A Book About Me!

Puberty during the Tweener Years

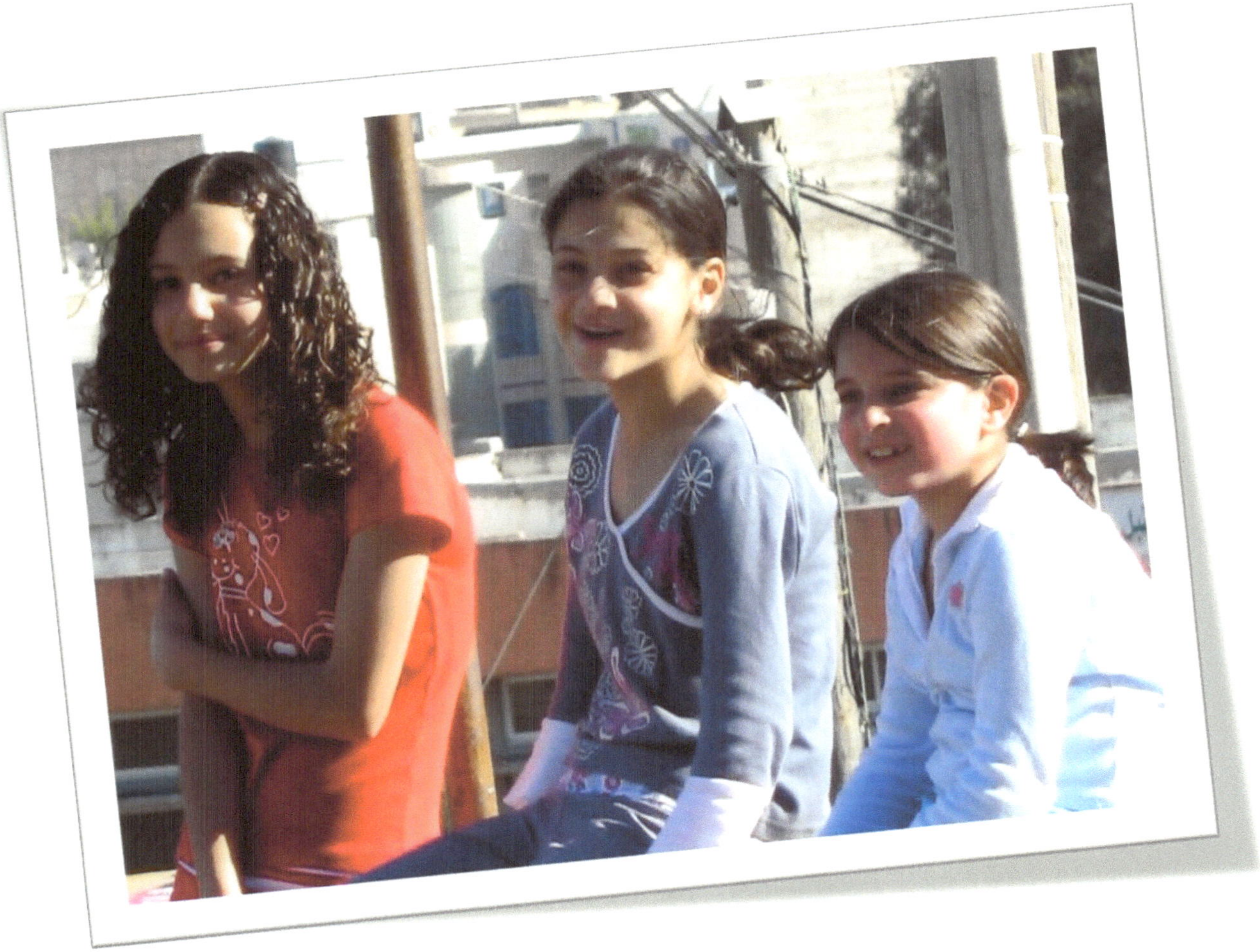

Table of Content

A Book About Me!

Between **0 to 2 years old**, you became a bouncing baby girl. At this stage, you learned how to sit up, began to point at objects, recognize people; but most of all, you learned how to recognize me – your mother. During your next stage in life, the toddler/preschool years (**2-5 years old**), you mastered walking, running, and you learned how to talk. Suddenly, you became "Ms. Independent."

PASTE A
TODDLER PICTURE

It was so difficult to stop you from trying to do everything on your own, especially putting on your clothes correctly. The good news, it was time for you to start your educational career. You were introduced to colors, shapes, numbers, and letters; but most of all, you were introduced to the outside world.

Adolescent – The Tweener Years

After years went by, your body began to develop and you began to see the world from a different point of view. I was no longer the center of your universe, and having friends became a huge part of your life. This is the time in which you began to bump heads with me and other adults. You would hear me say, "Fix your attitude;" "don't you roll your eyes at me;" and "stop acting like a baby!" Well, little do you know, you have entered into your **tweener years**.

PASTE A SCHOOL AGE PICTURE

A tweener is a young girl or boy between the ages of 10 to 12. This is the age group in which the majority of your peers are in middle school (grades 5 to 8). Your physical appearances and social development are caught between a young girl and a young woman. This book will teach you what to expect before you become a teenager (13 to 19 years old); but most of all, a young lady. In addition, you will learn what makes you different from a boy and how to properly take care of your body. So let's begin!

Puberty

Puberty is the stage of development in which your body leaves childhood and enters into womanhood. During this time in your life, your body will begin to change physically on the inside as well as the outside.

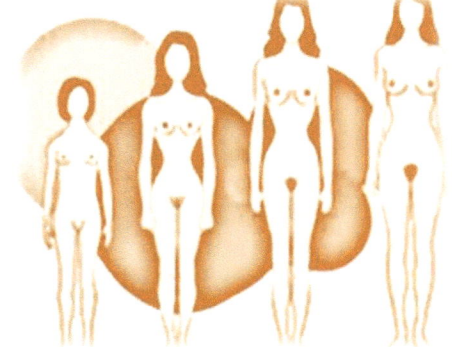

Don't worry, this is a normal process and it happens to every girl. There are several signs that your body is developing into a mature young lady such as your chest will begin to hurt and your nipples will become enlarge. You will also notice body hair under your armpits and hair on top of your vagina. Hair that grows on top of your vagina is called, **pubic hair**.

Once you begin puberty, it is a time to learn how to properly take care of your body – **hygiene**. In addition, this is the time when you should start

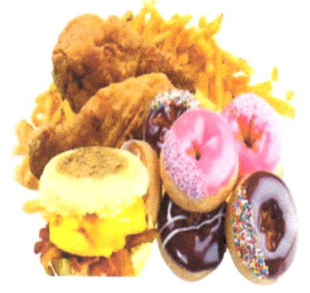

developing healthy eating habits in order to have beautiful skin, less stress, and avoid **acne** (pimples and blackheads). Pimples and blackheads are tiny little grease bumps that will appear during your tweener years. Acne will show up on your face, nose, chest, and back. The more junk food you eat, more likely acne will appear. However, the most noticeable change that will let you know that you are turning into a woman is having a **menstrual cycle** or better known as a **period**. Before we talk about having a period, let's talk about some additional changes that will occur in your tweener years.

During your adolescent years, the outside of your body will continue to develop body hair (i.e. underarms, legs, arms, and your face), and your 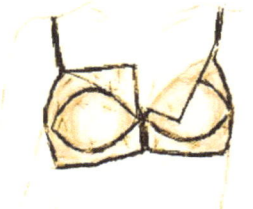 breast will continue to grow. Most tweeners start wearing a bra around 10 years old; sometimes earlier than that depending on the girl. Your vaginal area, which is also called your **pubic region,** prepares your body into womanhood.

Female Genital

The inside of your pubic area is made up of several parts: a vulva, vagina, cervix, uterus, two ovary sacs, and two fallopian tubes. The **vulva** is the skin on the outside of your vagina; it is the flappy skin that is covered in hair. It produces sweat glands and causes you to sweat; it will also cause you to have a musty odor. Your vulva area is very sensitive and must be protected and cleaned at all times. Cotton underwear is the best type of under garment to wear. It allows your vaginal area to breathe and minimize moisture; also, it protects your pubic area from germs and bacteria.

The vagina is located on the inside of the vulva that connects the cervix to the **uterus**. The **uterus** or sometimes called the **womb** is where a baby is developed. It's a muscle that looks like a pear and expand when a baby begins to grow. Each female is born with two **fallopian tubes** (oviducts) and two egg sacs, which are called **ovaries** (an ovum means one). Both sides of your uterus have an oviduct and are located on

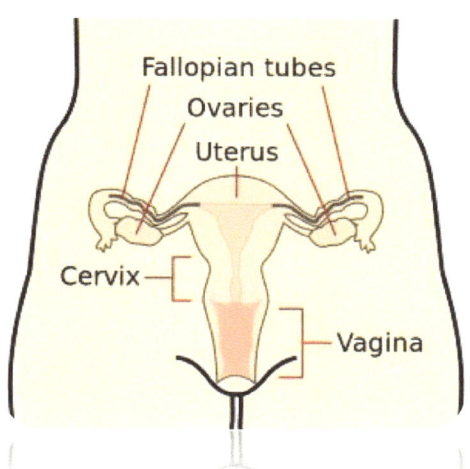

each side of the uterus. The fallopian tubes are used to fertilize an egg with a male sperm (girls have eggs and boys have sperm). If a sperm does not fertilize the egg, than it will travel down the fallopian tube and disintegrate or crumble. An egg that is not fertilized will cause you to have a menstrual cycle – a **blood flow**.

Before we began to discuss your period, you need to know about a leaky yellow fluid that shows up on your underwear before you begin a 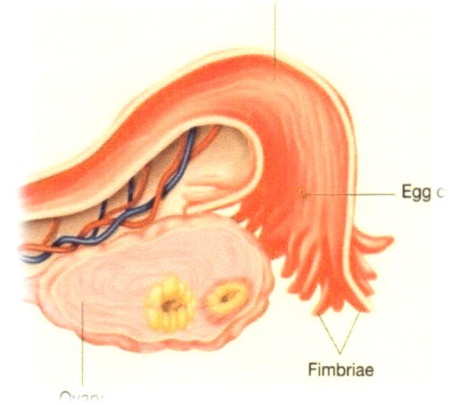 blood flow; it is called a **vaginal discharge**. A vaginal discharge is a yellowish fluid that comes out of the vagina. It is a fluid of white blood cells that kills bacteria and germs that grows inside of your body. Most likely, this fluid will turn white and should not leave a bad smell. This is a sign that you are about to start a period. If the fluid becomes a thick white discharge, looks like cottage cheese, and begins to itch, make sure you talk to me, or a health professional to obtain some type of medication. Now we can talk about having a period.

Menstrual Cycle

A woman is born with hundreds of immature eggs. Each egg is called an ovum and stored inside your ovary sacs until they become mature. Each month an egg is released into the fallopian tube; if fertilization does not happen, the egg will continue down the fallopian tube and dissolved into the uterus along with blood and dead uterine tissue.

Every 28 days, you will have a menstrual cycle; most girls start their period around the same time that their mother began theirs. Around the first 14 days of an average cycle, one of your ovaries will release an egg that will travel inside your fallopian tube; this stage is called **ovulation, or fertile time**. Ovulation is the time when a woman or girl can get pregnant by a male's sperm. If pregnancy does not occur, then the egg will dissolve into the uterus and your menstrual cycle will begin.

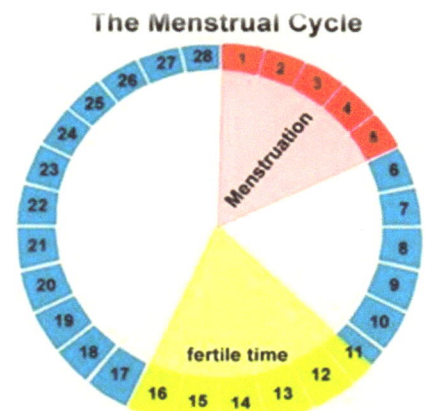

The first time you get your period, most likely it will be a very light red color or a brown sticky stain that will appear in your underwear. A period can last between 2 to 7 days depending on the girl. After having your second period, you should count the next 14 days before your next cycle begins, so that you can prepare to have personal hygienic products on hand. Some girls are excited when they began their period; others dread the day it comes. Cramps, mood swings, and severe pain can cause discomfort when you began your menstrual cycle. Some girls have really bad cramps, which can cause them to take medication or become very ill.

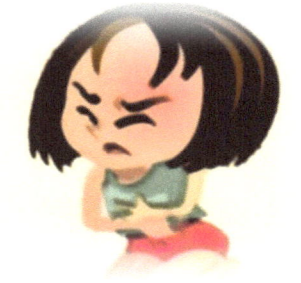 If you are experiencing really bad cramps or pain that causes you to become sick, make sure you tell me so that I can give you something to relieve some of the discomfort. Finally, there are several facts you should know before you start or when you are on your cycle:

- Most girls experience mood swings or become very emotional before or during their cycle; it is called, **Pre-Menstrual Syndrome (PMS)**. This will be discussed later.

- Blood should stop flowing if you decide to take a bath or go swimming.

- You can play sports if you desire; just bring extra pads.

- You are not considered dirty when you are on your period.

Remember, having a menstrual cycle is a normal process and it is a way that your body cleanses itself; so don't feel ashamed or become embarrass. Your body is letting you know that you have now entered into womanhood. Now, let's talk about how to properly take care of your body.

Proper Care of Your Body – Hygiene

Musk

As your body begins to develop and grow, you must learn how to properly take care of it. Once you start developing hair under your arms, you need to start wearing deodorant or antiperspirant. What cause your body to smell is bacteria that your body produces from your sweat glands; it's called, **musk**. Antiperspirant is used to keep you from sweating and deodorant helps to cover up the smell. Many people do not like to use

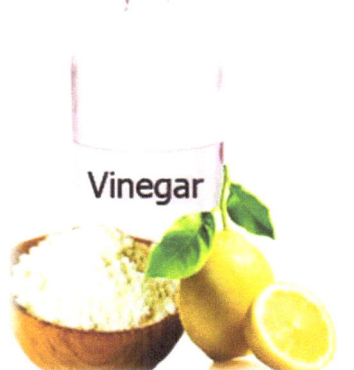

antiperspirant becomes of some of the active ingredients that can cause harm to your body. However, there are many **natural remedies** you can use to stop underarm odor. Apple cider vinegar, white vinegar, and Witch Hazel can reduce musk. In addition, baking soda and corn starch can absorb sweat and kill bacteria under your armpits as well.

Feminine Products

The most important way to keep your body clean or feeling fresh, particularly if you are on your period is soap and water. Soap and water is the best cleanser for your body. While you are on your period, you should change your pad frequently. This will help you to stay fresh and cause you to have fewer odors. I would suggest that you carry a personal hygiene kit when you are out and about. A personal hygiene kit should contain at least two sanitary napkins, 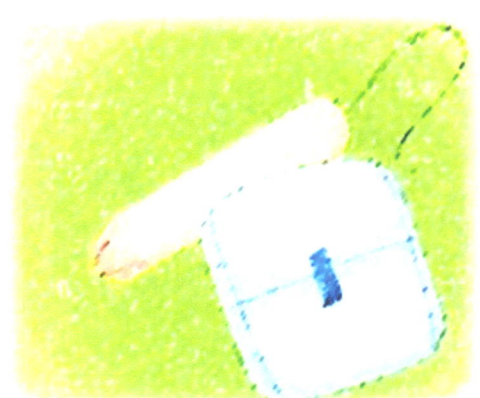 feminine hygiene wipes, a plastic bag, and an extra pair of underwear just in case the one that you are wearing becomes soiled.

Many teenage girls use tampons; a tampon is inserted inside of the vagina and absorbs the blood before it comes out of your body. However, many moms and health professionals do not recommend tampons for young girls because it can cause **Toxic Shock Syndrome (TSS)**. TSS is a dangerous infection, which can cause harmful bacteria to grow inside of your body and can cause you to become ill. Always talk to me or a health professional before you buy any type of personal hygiene products.

Lastly, to properly dispose of your soiled feminine napkin, roll the napkin in toilet paper tightly, and throw it away. I would recommend putting it into a small paper or plastic bag before disposal. But whatever you do, do not flush soiled pads or tampons down the toilet; it can clog up a drain.

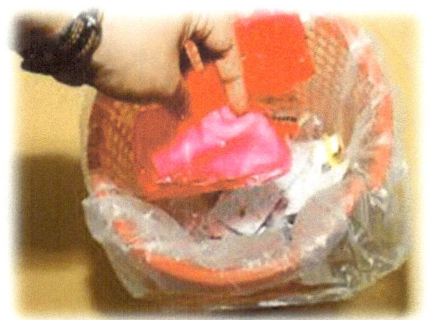

There are many products in the store to keep your vaginal area clean and fresh. Feminine sprays and vaginal wipes keep the outside of your pubic area clean. There are also feminine products that you can use to keep the inside of the vagina clean such as a **douche** (doosh). However, many health care professionals do not recommend using a douche because it can cause vaginal infections. If you decide that you would like to use a douche, make sure you to talk to me or a health care worker to learn what type of products to purchase, and how to properly use it.

Pre-Menstrual Syndrome (PMS)

Okay, before I end this book, I have to tell you that you might become a little crazy, mean, and emotional before or during your time of the month. Remember earlier, when I mentioned **Pre-Menstrual Syndrome (PMS)**? PMS is the cause of you having an attitude;

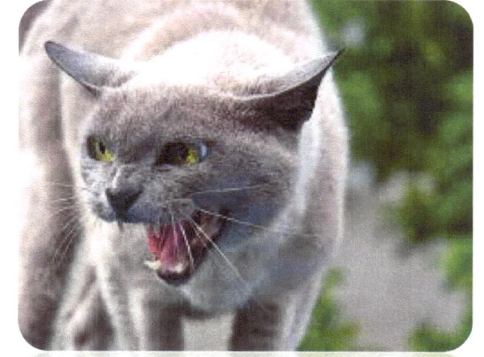

sometimes being mean; overly sensitive; and sometimes just feeling yucky. During your cycle, hormones inside your body are going to go up and down and cause you to have many mood

swings. Just relax, it is not going to last forever. My suggestion is to go exercise, or do something fun. Make sure you eat the right foods, drink lots of water, and get plenty of rest. And most of all,

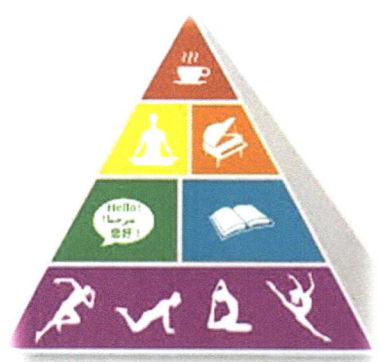

give yourself a time-out. Find out things that will help you get over your mood swings such as exercising, reading a good book, or meditation. Most likely, you are going to say sorry to a lot of people.

Oh! There is one last thing to talk about before I end this book –

weight gain. Before you begin your cycle, your body will

become bloated (retain water) and cause you to

gain weight, especially around your waist area.

Do not get depress when you look into the mirror.

You are going to realize that your favorite clothes will

not look good on you, or fit just right. Do not think that you are gaining

weight or you need to go on a diet. Just remember, the bloating will go

away and your body will return back to normal.

Conclusion

In nature, almost everything that produces life is called a female. A prominent female known throughout the world is **Mother Nature**. 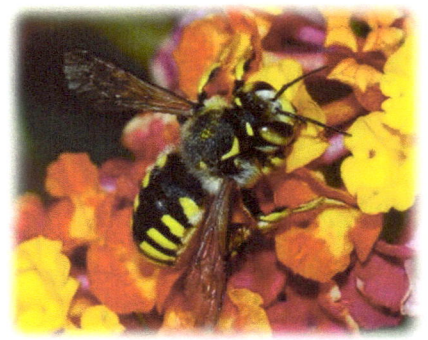 Mother Nature produces life and keeps the world looking beautiful. And yes, even she has a cycle. Her cycle is called the four seasons – winter, spring, summer, and fall. And finally, let's not forget our planet, who is also called by many people, particularly Native Americans, **Mother Earth**.

I know you might be thinking, "Good grief; this is a lot of work just to become a woman." Well, let me tell you, it is! But that's what makes you special! When God created female, He made you strong and courageous. He gave the woman a very special job liken unto Himself. Let's break down the word **FEMALE**. According to the Merriam Webster Dictionary, **FE** means **iron**. It is the chemical symbol used in chemistry that represents the strongest element in the world – iron. Therefore, it is not hard to believe that God made you into an iron male – FEMALE (smile).

26
Fe
55.845

The Creator made you close to Himself. You need to know that when God created the woman, He made us to be strong and powerful; but most of all, He made you to reflect the beauty of Himself. That is why it is so important to keep your body clean mentally (your thoughts), physically, and emotionally.

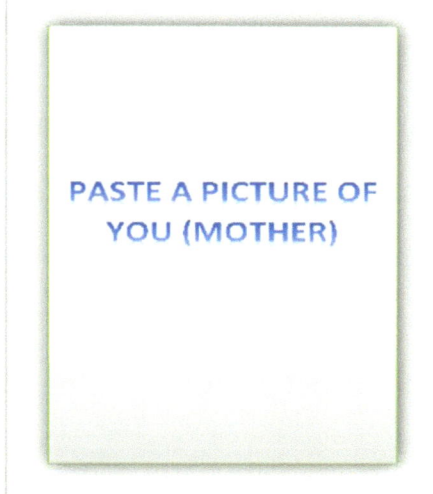

Always remember: a woman's body is made to produce and give life; your body is considered sacred (being holy) in the eyes of God. Not only is your body designed to bring life into the world, it is also made to give love. These are special reasons why you should keep your body clean and safe from harm. Also, be careful of what you put inside your body. Smoking, drinking alcohol, and eating a lot of bad foods (i.e. junk food), will cause your body to have health problems, terrible skin, and sometimes a bad attitude. Being a girl comes a lot a responsibility. However, if you take care of your body while you are young, you will blossom into a beautiful young woman like me.

Love Always

Mom

Glossary

1. **Acne** – Acne is a skin condition that shows up as different types of bumps (i.e. whiteheads), blackheads, and pimples (red bumps).

2. **Cervix** – The narrow neck-like passage forming the lower end of the uterus.

3. **Fallopian Tubes** – A pair of tubes located inside of female that allows eggs to travel from the ovaries to the uterus.

4. **Hygiene** – A practice to maintain health and preventing disease, especially through cleanliness.

5. **Menstrual Cycle** – The process of ovulation and menstruation in females.

6. **Ovaries** – A pair of female reproductive organ in which ova or eggs are produced.

7. **Puberty** – The period during which adolescents reach sexual maturity and become capable of reproduction.

8. **Uterus (Womb)** - The organ in the lower body of a woman or female animal where babies are developed

9. **Vulva** - A female's external genitals.

10. **Vagina** - The muscular tube leading from the external genitals to the cervix of the uterus in women and in most female mammals.

What's Happening to Me?

At the age of 10, my body: _____

_____
_____
_____
_____
_____
_____
_____

At the age of 11, my body: _____

_____
_____
_____
_____
_____
_____
_____

At the age of 12, my body: _____

_____
_____
_____
_____
_____
_____
_____

At the age of 13, my body: _____

_____
_____
_____
_____
_____
_____
_____

At the age of 14, my body: _____

_____
_____
_____
_____
_____
_____
_____

At the age of 15, my body: _____

_____
_____
_____
_____
_____
_____
_____

Taking Care of Yourself

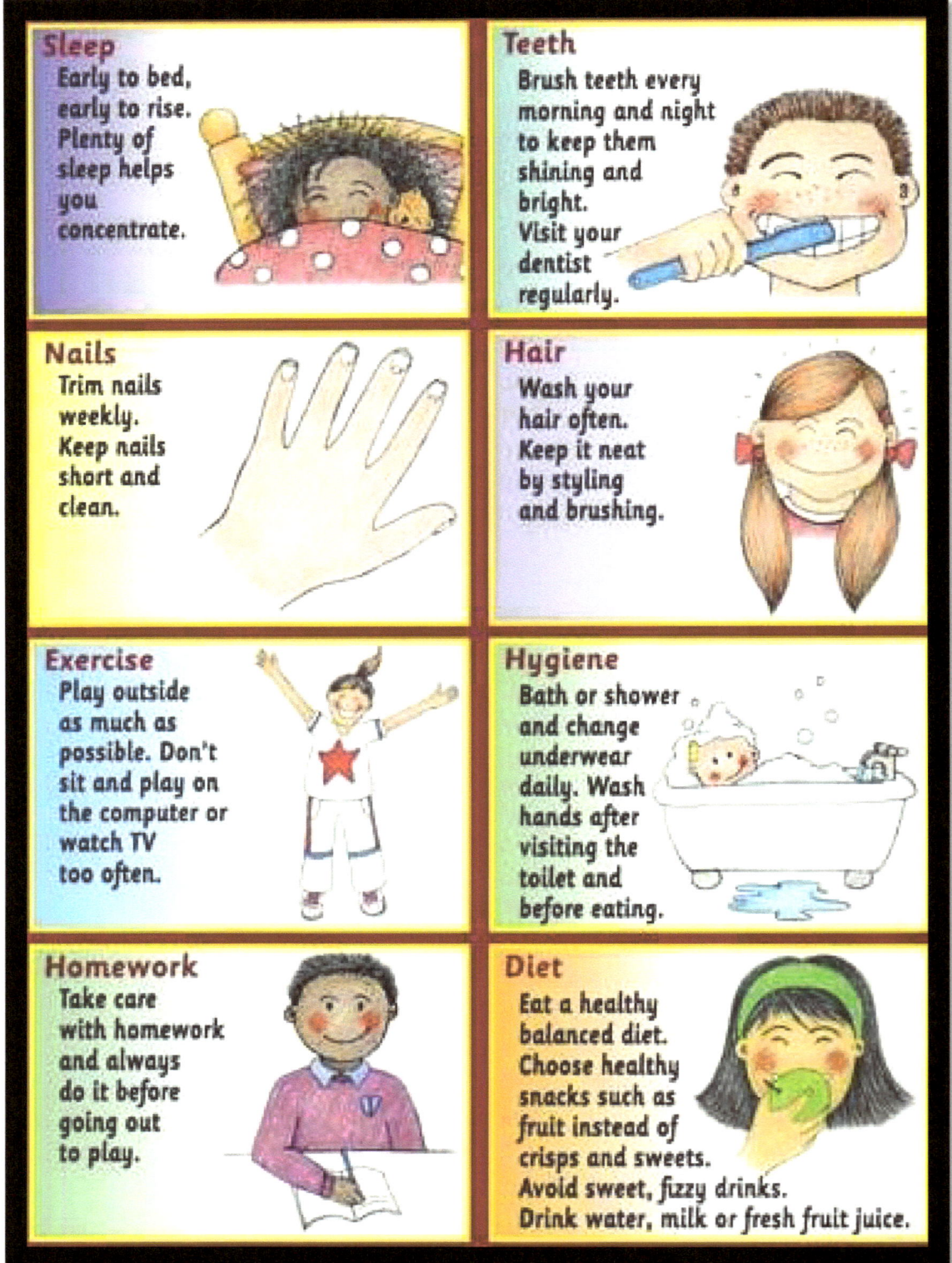

Sleep
Early to bed, early to rise. Plenty of sleep helps you concentrate.

Teeth
Brush teeth every morning and night to keep them shining and bright. Visit your dentist regularly.

Nails
Trim nails weekly. Keep nails short and clean.

Hair
Wash your hair often. Keep it neat by styling and brushing.

Exercise
Play outside as much as possible. Don't sit and play on the computer or watch TV too often.

Hygiene
Bath or shower and change underwear daily. Wash hands after visiting the toilet and before eating.

Homework
Take care with homework and always do it before going out to play.

Diet
Eat a healthy balanced diet. Choose healthy snacks such as fruit instead of crisps and sweets. Avoid sweet, fizzy drinks. Drink water, milk or fresh fruit juice.

Monthly Journal

I began my menstrual cycle on
Date: _____
I experienced: _____

_____

_____

_____

I began my menstrual cycle on
Date: _____
I experienced: _____

_____

_____

_____

I began my menstrual cycle on
Date: _____
I experienced: _____

_____

_____

_____

I began my menstrual cycle on
Date: _____
I experienced: _____

_____

_____

_____

I began my menstrual cycle on
Date: _____
I experienced: _____

_____

_____

_____

I began my menstrual cycle on
Date: _____
I experienced: _____

_____

_____

_____

I began my menstrual cycle on
Date: _____
I experienced: _____

_____

_____

_____

I began my menstrual cycle on
Date: _____
I experienced: _____

_____

_____

_____

I began my menstrual cycle on
Date: _____
I experienced: _____

_____

_____

_____

I began my menstrual cycle on
Date: _____
I experienced: _____

_____

_____

_____

I began my menstrual cycle on
Date: _____
I experienced: _____

_____

_____

_____

I began my menstrual cycle on
Date: _____
I experienced: _____

_____

_____

_____

I began my menstrual cycle on
Date: _____
I experienced: _____

_____

_____

_____

I began my menstrual cycle on
Date: _____
I experienced: _____

_____

_____

_____

I began my menstrual cycle on
Date: _____
I experienced: _____

_____

_____

_____

I began my menstrual cycle on
Date: _____
I experienced: _____

_____

_____

_____

A Story About Me

I was told, when I was little _____

_____

_____

_____

_____

_____

_____

As I got older_____

_____

_____

_____

_____

In my family, there is _____

_____

_____

_____

I go to worship at _____

I like to go because _____

The reason why I don't like to go _____

I go to school at _____

_____

_____

_____

My favorite subject is _____

The reason why it is my favorite subject_____

_____

_____

_____

My friends' are_____

_____

However, my best friend (s) _____

_____

_____

_____

My favorite things I like to do_____

_____

The reason why_____

_____

_____

_____

My favorite foods are _____

_____

_____

_____

_____

My favorite holiday is _____

The reason why it is my favorite _____

_____

_____

I will never forget the day when I had so much fun _____

_____

_____

_____

_____

One of my saddest memories was _____

_____

_____

_____

_____

I know that I am special because _____

_____

_____

_____

_____

When I get older, I would like to be _____

_____

_____

_____

_____

The reason why _____

_____

_____

_____

_____

So far; all of these things that has happened to me, is making me into a beautiful, young lady who I am growing up to be!

THE END

www.ingramcontent.com/pod-product-compliance
Lightning Source LLC
Chambersburg PA
CBHW060818290526
45792CB00005BB/1713